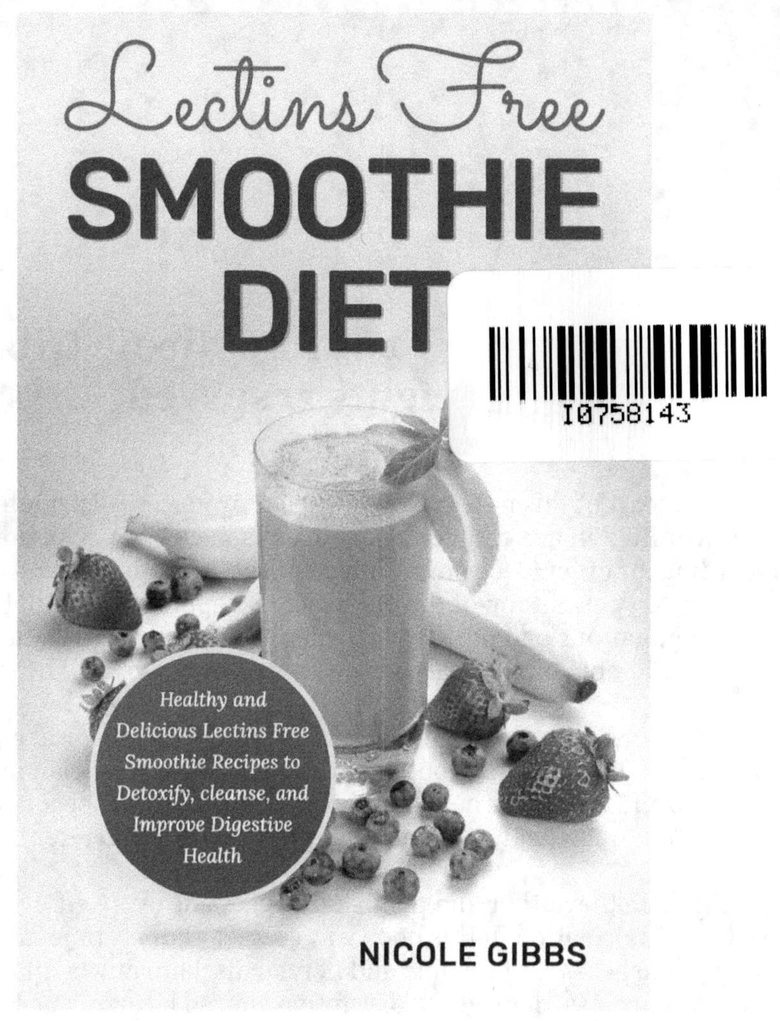

Lectins Free Smoothie Diet

Healthy and Delicious Lectins Free Smoothie Recipes to Detoxify, Cleanse, and Improve Digestive Health

Dedication

I dedicate this book to help anyone who is willing to meet their individual health needs and wellness goals by educating them to make better food choices to approach better health. I truly hope you take advantage of the knowledge and experience this book has to offer to help you improve your health.

Table of Content

Introduction

For most of us, we see vegetables and think that they're automatically healthy.

But, some foods, especially those with dairy, legumes and nightshades, and even grains aren't good for you either.

Lectins can cause harm to the body in different ways, and it's important to understand what they can do for you.

There are ways to make foods devoid of lectins, and it's important to look into this as well.

Here, we'll go over what the lectins-free diet is, and also include some amazing smoothies for you to try!

Your body doesn't need a bunch of lectins. In fact, it's better if they don't get this. You should try to eliminate these foods rich in lectins, so that you can have a happy, healthy existence.

In this book, we'll go over how to eat properly despite the presence of lectins in a diet, and what exactly you need to do in order to begin the lectin-free diet, including what should be eaten, what shouldn't, and any concerns associated with lectins that you need to watch out for.

By the end of this, you'll be able to easily and effectively take care of your body, and have less lectins than before. Lectins can cause a lot of issues with your gut health and inflammation, but we'll go over all of that in the ensuing chapters.

Chapter 1
The True Meaning of Lectins

First, let's go over what lectins are. While they are in many nutritious foods, they actually can cause a lot of problems, especially with gut health.

Some nutrition experts have found that this protein can also cause some very detrimental problems, including harming the immune system, increasing inflammation, and increasing your risk for chronic diseases and autoimmune issues.

Lectin-rich foods are not bad for you completely, but for some people, it can impact the gut health of the body. Here, we'll go over what the lectins are, why it's important to understand, and what the lectins-free diet entails.

What is the Lectins-Free Diet?

First let's talk about what lectins are. Of course the diet will involve reducing or eliminating the intake of lectins.

But why should you avoid having these?

Lectins are essentially a group of proteins that are seen primarily in legumes and grains. They perform a lot of different bodily functions, including your immune system and improving your blood protein levels.

However, the problem is most of us don't eat the proper amount of lectins. Having too much can cause a lot of problems, particularly in your gut.

Vomiting, bowel issues, diarrhea, and other gut health problems can be a big part of it. We'll go over what other issues come from consuming too many lectins later on.

The diet focuses primarily on reducing the lectins in your diet. You can of course go cold turkey with this, but it's best if you slowly reduce this. If you're sensitive to eliminating foods, this can be a whole lot more beneficial.

It does eliminate a lot of nutrient-dense foods however, since a lot of them have lectins. For example, beans are eliminated in a lot of cases, although they can be healthy for you.

If you cook some of the lectin-rich foods that are out there, such as beans in water, this does reduce the lectins in there. This makes them safer for consumption.

Some foods such as nuts and peanuts aren't affected by cooking though. So you should make sure that you don't consume too much of it.

You can eat foods with it, so long as they're destroyed before consumption as well.

The goal of this is to help reduce inflammation and improper gut health in the body,

Are Lectins bad for your health?

As we've said before, these proteins are bound to carbs, and they are in a lot of our foods. Plant and animal products are filled with this.

While there isn't a ton of research on the effects of this to fully conclude that they're bad for everyone, too much of this can cause problems.

There are some studies which say this is what's called an antinutrient. This means that it can impact how your body takes in nutrients from foods. Other studies have found that lectins can affect people who have a sensitive digestive system, or who experience distress on a gastrointestinal level.

Lectins can also impact the gut health of your body and how it absorbs nutrients. This can increase inflammation and reduce the secretion of acids.

This can cause long-term problems and impacts down the line, so; it's important to make sure that if you consume them, you don't have too many. Just like with anything, too much of something can be a problem.

The issue with lectins though is that they're present in food that is good for you. Usually, they are in foods that have a ton of vitamins, antioxidants, and some minerals which are good for the body. But for those with sensitive digestion, this could wreak havoc on your body too.

This can in some cases bind to the membranes of your digestive system, and from there, cause metabolism concerns and damage too. If you have a digestive condition such as IBS, or experience problems when consuming these foods it may be because of the lectins. If you've got a sensitive stomach, lectins can possibly irritate this too.

Ideally, you should avoid foods that cause problems in the body for you, so you should, if you do have these, use your discretion and if it's causing issues for you physically, then stop consuming them.

The Harmful Effects of Lectins

The problem with lectins is that they can cause issues with autoimmune concerns in the body. For example, if you have rheumatoid arthritis, this can play a part in flaring it up. Autoimmune conditions and chronic pain do get flared up if you consume too many lectins, since the gut and the immune health are intimately connected.

Having too many lectins can also of course, cause digestive issues. Have you ever had beans that weren't cooked and suddenly felt like you were going to throw up, or felt sick? That's because you had too many lectins, and if you have a sensitive stomach, it can cause gastroenteritis, which can flare up digestive symptoms and in some cases may cause lectin poisoning too. Since it is an antinutrient too, it can also cause issues with absorption and digestion of foods, causing more nutritional deficiencies to be a major problem.

Lectins can be toxic for the body too. Some lectins have different effects on the body. While some of them are not as bad for you, there are those that are from castor beans which can be toxic for the body. This of course, manifests itself in diarrhea and vomiting after eating a little.

If you've gotten sick after eating raw or undercooked beans, chances are that's because of the lectin in the body. Cooking beans does help make them less toxic, and much safer to eat. However, don't' slow cook the beans.

I can possibly cause permanent damage to the intestines as well. Because it can stop digestion and absorbing nutrients, this can stop a part of the digestive system over time. If you eat a ton of these over a long period, this can happen. However, the studies on this are still limited, so if you do already have issues with absorbing nutrients, it's important to not irritate this further.

Finally, the biggest downside associated with this is inflammation, particularly digestive inflammation. But this can impact a lot of the inflammation in the body, causing autoimmune conditions to flare up over time.

One thing that can happen with too many lectins is that it can permanently damage the gut wall, which causes leaky gut. Leaky gut causes permeability issues, which cause substances to leak into your bloodstream itself. This means that inflammatory conditions can cause inflammation through the entire body in a lot of cases.

So yes, too many lectins causes major issues, from gut health concerns to toxicity, but luckily, the lectins-free diet is an option to consider.

What are the worst veggies for Your Gut?

The worst ones for your gut health are nightshades and legumes, but let's get a little more specific.

Dates are actually one of the worst. They have sulfites in them, which causes diarrhea, gas, bloating, nausea, and even asthma too. They aren't good for sensitive stomachs, and too much fiber can cause irritability in the gut too.

Onions aren't good for your gut either. While they're great for improving immunity, too much of this causes major gut health issues, and if you have them with garlic, it gets worse. It can cause cramping, bloating, and for those with sensitive digestions, it can cause these symptoms to really flare up.

Brussels sprouts are probably one of the worst too, simply because of the fructans in it, which is fermented in your gut after you consume this. This can cause major abdominal issues, and it can be a big pain to deal with. Fully eliminating or cutting them out to smaller portions may be a valid option for you if you really love your sprouts.

Asparagus is another one. There are a lot of fructans in this, and it's one of the worst for gut health. For those who have pre-existing gut health issues such as IBS, this can cause the symptoms to get way worse. It can also impact the colon too, if you're not sure about cutting it out, do so for a bit and see what happens next.

Finally, there is mushrooms, which causes gut irritation due to the sugar alcohol in it. You may notice that it is irritating you immensely, so you may want to cut out the mushrooms if you notice it being too much for your gut health.

What to Eat on a Lectin-Free Diet

The thing is, almost all plants and animals have lectins in them. However, some are worse than others, and won't' totally impact your gut health in a bad way.

Some of the things to eat on this diet do include:

-Apples
-Arugula
-Beets
-Blueberries

-Broccoli
-Cabbage
-Artichokes
-Asparagus
-Blackberries
-Bok choy
-Carrots
-Celery
-Chives
-Cranberries
-Leafy greens
-Lemons
-Okra
-Cauliflower
-Cherries
-Collars
-Kale
-Leeks
-Oranges
-Radishes
-Scallions
-Sweet potatoes
-Pumpkins
-Raspberries
-Strawberries
-Swiss chard

You can also have some animal protein including fish, chicken, beef, and eggs, but you should be wary about this.

As for fats, you should have healthier fats such as those in butter, avocados, and also olive oil too

You can have some nuts on this, including pecans, pine nuts, flax and hemp seeds, and some brazil nuts too

However, you should be careful about stuff that contains larger amounts of lectin, since that of course can impact your gut health in the worst of ways.

What not to eat on a Lectin-Free Diet

The foods that you need to avoid the most include:

-Legumes such as peanuts, lentils, chickpeas, and beans. Even if they're soaked in water they have a lot of high levels of lectins

-Nightshades including tomatoes, goji berries, eggplants, peppers, and potatoes

-Anything with peanut in it, so no peanut butter or oil

-Most dairy products

-All grains that have a grain or some flour in them, which does include crackers, cakes, and breads

-Baked goods of any kinds

All of these do have lectins in it that are much higher than the others. While it is hard to avoid lectins, the amount of these is far more than one thinks, and it can be detrimental.

While cooking does fix this for a couple of them, such as the legumes, it doesn't for the rest.

Low Lectin Foods to Enjoy!

The best low-lectin foods that you can enjoy include the following:

-Leafy greens, especially spinach
-Celery
-Pasture-raised meats
-Sweet potatoes that are cooked
-Avocadoes
-Any oils that are healthy, including olive and extra-virgin olive oils

In general, you want to avoid most of the foods that are listed as bad for you, and you should work to slowly reduce this, or eliminate them fully.

If you do have a bad gut, consider trying to avoid these first, and then slowly introduce and see how this makes you feel after that's introduced completely.

Chapter 2
Thriving on a Lectins-Free Diet

So how do you thrive on this?

The problem with the lectin-free diet is that it's incredibly restrictive, so you need to make sure that you're eating enough nutrients in the foods that you consume.

The problem is, a lot of the foods which are eliminated contain large amounts of fiber. Fiber is good for your gut health, but for those with gut issues including IBS, this can impact how your gut absorbs it. There are a few things that you should do before you start on this diet.

First, you need to make sure that you're getting enough fruits and veggies in order to compensate for the lack of fiber that you have otherwise. Having fruits that are high in fiber to compensate for this is good, and a lot of the low-lectin foods suggested contain a lot of vitamins, minerals, and antioxidants too.

Another thing to consider is supplements. If you plan to do this to change your gut health, you'll want to make sure that you have a few supplements. For starters, a fiber supplement may be good too, especially if you're not getting enough fiber.

You also may want to consider a protein supplement if that's what you're lacking. In general, a supplement to help compensate for what you lack is important, so make sure that you do this, especially when you're looking to have lectin content that's effective and easy.

Replenishing your Kitchen with Lectin-free Foods

So what's the best way to replenish the kitchen with these foods?

Well, first and foremost, you may want to try the elimination diet. This is where you remove foods and see if the symptoms get better. Start by removing foods high in lectins such as grains and dairy, and see how you feel over time. If the source is lectins, remove this and start to replace.

Create a weekly grocery list and make sure that you have this in place. When you go to the store, get this, and from there, eat that. We'll go over meal prep later on, but having a grocery list on hand to start your diet is important.

When replenishing your kitchen, don't just toss all of it away. You should make sure to eliminate and see if that's what's causing the flare-ups. You may discover that you don't have issues with nightshades, but you have issues when consuming dairy.

If you're going to keep some of the foods to avoid around, try to see if you can cook the lectin out of it. Peanuts of course can't have the lectin cooked out but beans of all kinds can have the lectin reduced.

And remember that not all foods with lectins are bad. A lot of them contain valuable antioxidants and such. The best thing for you to do at that point is to choose and find the ones that cause trouble.

You also can slowly integrate this too. You don't have to do it right away, but slowly eliminating these items to live a truly lectin-free lifestyle is a good idea.

Easy and Fast Strategies for Success

Here are a few simple strategies to truly benefit from the lectin-free diet.
For starters, you'll want to have a meal plan, but also take into consideration the idea of the elimination diet to determine if it's a food allergy or something else.

If you're looking to still eat grains and beans, consider fermenting or sprouting them. This takes a little bit longer to prepare, but it does reduce the amount of lectin in the food as well before you eat it.

Along with that, get into the habit of soaking and then boiling your beans to help with reducing this.

When it comes to eating meals, some of the best ways are through shakes, but it's good to have a plan for the week. We'll go over why that is in the next section, but a plan for your meals is important, so you can make sure you're getting enough calories and nutrients.

Speaking of calories, while this diet isn't used for weight loss, it can potentially help with this. However, if you find that you're not eating enough, you should consider looking for different ways to incorporate more calories and nutrients into this.

And of course, you shouldn't be afraid to have a supplement. We'll go over what that is later on.

Finally, you should consult your dietician or doctor so that you can make sure that you're getting the nutrients that you need every single day. This is important, because a lot of people start this diet and then get into health issues from the lack of nutrients. By consulting your doctor and ensuring that you get something good for you, you'll be able to with this have a good means to really take care of yourself, and really help you get the most that you can out of this.

Don't be afraid to cook your foods or add to your smoothies some fun little additives, which we'll go over in chapter 3.

Planning your Weekly Meal Plans

Now the next big thing to do when you're using this diet, is meal plans., specifically, weekly meal plans.
Why is that? **It's because you want to make sure you do the following:**

-Buy the foods that you need without overspending
-Have a plan for what to eat
-It offers more control over your diet
-It also prevents you from slipping

Even just a general idea of the meal plan is important. Having a solid understanding of what you're going to eat is good.

That way, you can also track whether or not something is beneficial to you, and whether or not you'll need to eliminate it from the diet or not.

This also helps you plan so that you're eating foods that you can enjoy. The biggest problem with diets is the fact that they usually involve foods being eaten countless times. Having the same meal multiple days in a row gets boring, and you can't simply just do that. Instead, you want to make sure that you eat the proper foods, take the initiative to eat right, and at the end of it, really improve your health and wellness.

Meal planning puts you in control, so it's recommended to do.

Guide to Buying Produce and Whole Foods

When buying produce, make sure it's not a legume, nightshade, or anything with high levels of lectins. So of course, beans and lentils should be avoided.

You can have sweet potatoes so long as they're cooked, but you should avoid potatoes. Even if they are cooked, you will still have high amounts of lectins.

If you're buying any sorts of animal products, you want to make sure that they're grass-fed or organic meats and proteins. You should make sure they aren't pumped with hormones or anything else, since it then defeats the purpose of buying the products for the diet.

When it comes to grains, you should avoid anything that's unable to be fermented. All processed grains and baked goods should be avoided too.

When shopping, you should shop around the perimeter, and avoid of course the inner parts of the aisles, which is usually where all the processed foods go.

When it comes to fruits and veggies, you can also flavor them with some herbs and spices too. I'd suggest if you're looking for something good for your foods, you should get some species and herbs, put them in there, and have them.

All in all, you should make sure that you follow the meal plan that you have, and only buy for that meal plan. Get the fruits and veggies that you know that you'll eat, and avoid those with large amounts of lectins.

As for dairy, you should avoid this, especially if you're doing elimination to see where the problem is.

Remember that not all lectins are bad for you. In fact, some of the healthiest foods have these, but the fact of the matter is simple. Make sure that you're not eating too many, and having some precaution when choosing the different kinds of foods that you'd like to eat.

Chapter 3
Lectins-Free Smoothies

One way to do the lectins free diet is to make smoothies!

Lectins free smoothies are essentially smoothies that are made without lectins. It's simple, but incredibly effective.

There are a few reasons why lots of people will use smoothies instead of just cooking meals. While it does mean that you may need to consume more duet to the lack of chewing associated with smoothies, this also supplies nutrients quickly and effectively.

That's why a lot of people like to have lectins-free smoothies. We'll go over here what lectins-free smoothies are, and the benefits of a smoothie diet.

Why Smoothies are the best method for this Diet

The lectins free diet involves eating lots of plants and plant food. There are a lot of benefits associated with drinking smoothies. They're not only a cool drink, but they're also good for you to really get the most out of your diet.

For starters, they do help you feel full. If you're looking to lose weight while also improving your gut health, you'll be able to have these as alternatives. The fruits and veggies within this are good for staying full for a longer period of time.

They also help with cravings. Smoothies contain a variety of nutrients which are necessary to help keep you away from junk food consumption. The proteins within this will help with that too, and the variety of nutrients even in lectins free smoothies are good for you.

But probably one of the biggest benefits is what it does to your gut health. Smoothies are wonderful for aiding indigestion. Most of the smoothies on the lectins free diet are plant-based smoothies that contain a lot of vitamins and some minerals to help with digestion. You can have that shot directly into your gut, and help with aiding digestion. This is really good because it also contains fiber too. While you're not breaking it down, the fiber will be more direct to your system, allowing for multiple benefits as well.

And not just that, it also helps with the antioxidants too. When you do the lectins free diet with non-smoothie options, it can cause nutritional problems due to the lack of antioxidants. However with a smoothie, you can add little goodies to this. Matcha green powder is really good to help with many different diseases. Grapes and berries are good for this too, and you can even add some good sweet potatoes to help with this diet.

This in turn will help with your immunity too. Lots of the smoothies that we have on here contain a lot of great benefits that will help you directly, meaning that you don't need to jump through hoops to get the benefits. This is especially good for the lectins free diet.

With the lectins free diet, you're given a lot of foods which may be hard to cook with. But with a smoothie, it injects all of that straight into you, meaning that you'll get the benefits of this right away.

Benefits of the Smoothie Diet

Smoothies are great for a variety of reasons. The smoothie diet is pretty simple to follow.

The premise is simple: you consume most of your meals and foods through a smoothie, rather than of course, manually eating it.

This is really good for those of us who are on the go. I'm sure you don't want to sit around and do super excessive meal prep. But with the smoothies you have, you can make a few, pack them and put them in the fridge, and then have them for when you need them during the week. This is especially good for those of us who are not in the mood to cook a bunch of meals.

With the smoothie diet, you can have breakfast, lunch, and dinner smoothies, with small meals throughout this. But this gets the nutrients that you need directly, without needing to wait for them to digest. This gets the antioxidants and vitamins that you need right there, so it's all waiting for you.

Smoothies are also very simple to make. For those of us who aren't good at cooking, this is probably your best option. You can just throw it in the blender, add some fun additions, and then there you go.

That's another big part about smoothies. They're incredibly customizable. You don't need to be a master chef to make these right. Even if your knowledge of cooking is minimal, if you learn how to make smoothies and simply put them together to drink, this can offer a variety of health benefits.

And finally, they taste great too. A lot of people when they start diets don't like to do it because the foods get bland, boring, and unpalatable. Thankfully with smoothies, you simply throw them in, turn it on, let it pulsate, and then there you go! That's easy.

With all of this being said, there's a ton of benefits to smoothies, and a whole lot that you can do with smoothies, so make sure that you take the time to ensure that you'll get the most that you can out of them, no matter what.

Health Benefits of Using smoothies

Smoothies have a lot of health benefits to them as well, not just for providing the nutrients that you need either.

For starters, if you add certain supplements to this, it can really work its magic. But even if you don't, adding some fruits such as kiwis and bananas, can help with a variety of problems.

Sleep problems can be curbed with this. Adding calcium and magnesium can help with inducing sleep and improving your sleep patterns, so if you're looking to get better sleep so you're happy and healthy, this is definitely something for you to do.

Smoothies also are good for the outer appearance of your body too. Pumpkins and mangoes for example contain carotenoids. This is really good for your skin and complexion too, so if you want to take care of your skin and look great, this is a good way to do it.

This is liquid food, and it can be better for bodily breakdown as well. Since a lot of people use the lectin-free diet to aim with gut health, this can be easier on the gut, and will help with properly breaking down the body and improving it too!

You can also naturally detox the body every day too. Beets and papaya, along with trace amounts of garlic, can help with any toxins in the body. Since of course, you use this diet in order to help rid the toxins there, this can be great for detoxifying everything, and it can be good as well to start the day.

Finally, with a lot of the veggies and fruits that are in there, you can improve your brain health and memory as well. Being mentally alert and able to concentrate is benefitted by the ingredients in these. Adding coconut oil or even just some coconut milk as an alternative has a lot of omega-3 fatty acids, and this can help boost your brain power to work even better.

Smoothies are good for getting all of those nutrients that you know and love directly, and effectively, so it's no wonder why a lot of people enjoy smoothies! They're good, and they're good for you!

Why you Should add a Plant-Based Protein to Your Smoothie!

Some people like to add different supplements to their smoothies and that's a great thing.

Adding more antioxidants and vitamins to your smoothie is really good, simply because it gives you a whole lot more goodies all in one drink.

But one thing that you should consider adding more than anything else, is protein powder.

Protein powder is perfect for a smoothie.

Why is that? Well have you ever had a smoothie but then felt hungry a few minutes later? That's probably because you didn't have a protein supplement added to your smoothie.

By incorporating a protein powder, you'll have a meal that's more balanced, and way more filling.

This takes your regular smoothie and makes it something filling and something that tastes amazing.

Usually you just need a scoop to get it right, and one scoop can have up to 30 grams of protein in one scoop! It's pretty awesome, and it can help make any smoothie into something you can enjoy.

With the smoothies that we'll have listed, we'll be writing them like you're adding a scoop of a 20 grams of protein to this.

It will make the calories a bit higher for your average smoothie, but that's also taking into account the fact that you'll be fuller, and your meals will be more spread out.

You can also add other supplements too such as extra greens or matcha powder, but if nothing else, make sure you add protein.

With this being said, it's time to go over 30 amazing smoothies that you can enjoy, and some great ones not just for breakfast, but also for lunch and dinner too, all lectin-free!

Chapter 4
Lectins-Free Smoothie Recipes!

And here are 30 amazing recipes that work wonders for those looking to be lectin-free. They are simple to make, and are great for keeping you full during the day, and are also a good replacement option for meals.

If you are going to replace one meal with this, it is recommended to add a protein substitute for it. These smoothies are written without the addition, so when it comes to calories, just make sure to add the total for the protein substitute that you include in there.

10 Breakfast Lectins-Free Smoothie Recipes

Avocado Green Smoothie

The avocado smoothie. While this was popularized by artist Jason Mraz, this is a popular smoothie simply because of how good this tastes, and the amazing health benefits.

Ingredients:

- [ ] 1.5 cups of cold almond milk or coconut milk, unsweetened
- [ ] 1 banana, ripe
- [ ] 1 sliced apple
- [ ] 2 cups packed kale leaves
- [ ] 1 avocado, ripe
- [ ] 1 small stalk of chopped celery
- [ ] 1 piece of fresh, peeled ginger
- [ ] Ice cubes

Directions:

-Blend the milk beverage all together

-When it's smooth, you simply take it out and drink it. Serves two

Nutritional information:

Calories: 307

Protein: 5g
Carbs: 41g
Fiber: 12g
Fat: 17g
Sodium: 144 mg

The Perfect Beginner Green Smoothie

This is a great one because it has the fruit-to-veggie ratio, so it's perfect for those looking to have more green smoothies. You do notice the spinach in this, but the taste is mild, and it comes with nutrients, minerals, antioxidants, and all kinds of great stuff. It's even good for kids too

Ingredients:

- ☐　2 cups spinach
- ☐　1 cup pineapple
- ☐　1 cup mango
- ☐　2 cups water
- ☐　2 bananas

Directions:

-Put the leafy greens together and pack them.

-Add in the water and blend it till the leafy chunks disappear

-Add in the other ingredients and then blend this until smooth. Ideally, serve this in a mason jar

Nutritional information:

Calories: 220
Fat: 13g
Protein: 6g
Carbs: 33g
Sodium: 100 mg

Breakfast Green Smoothie Recipe

This is a great one for those of us who enjoy bananas, since that's the primary flavor of this. That, and it comes with a lot of lectins-free ingredients such as seeds of choice

Ingredients:

- ☐　1 cup frozen fruit of choice such as berries or bananas

- ☐ 1 cup almond or coconut milk
- ☐ 1 cup spinach or kale
- ☐ ½ tablespoon flax or chia seeds

Directions:

-Take the ingredients and put them in a blender.

-Start with ½ a cup of the milk and then add a bit more if you'd like something thicker

-Banana is the ideal one because it's got some amazing tastes to it, and really will give you a great touch

Nutritional information:

Calories: 146
Fat: 3g
Carbs: 30g
Fiber: 5g
Protein: 3g

Chard Avocado Breakfast Smoothie

This is an interesting one because it not only comes with the fruity touch of the banana and avocado, but it also comes with some healthy greens. People usually do a handful of chard, but if you're not a fan of that, you can substitute this with kale for best results.

Some like to also have this in a smoothie bowl, which is an alternative

Ingredients:

- ☐ ½ a ripe avocado
- ☐ ½ a cup of coconut milk
- ☐ 1 ripe banana
- ☐ 1 handful of greens of choice
- ☐ 1 cup ice

Directions:

-Take the banana and avocado, put it in the blender

-Add in the ice then the green parts

-Blend it till everything's blended

-You can add more coconut milk to enhance the texture of the smoothie

Nutritional information:

Calories: 145
Fat: 10g
Protein: 6g
Fiber: 13g
Carbs: 35g

Minty Breakfast Smoothie

Again, another tasty smoothie with some refreshing avocadoes, and this is a fun one that will stimulate your taste buds in all the right ways. That, and the refreshing taste of mint definitely adds a kicker to the fun smoothie

Ingredients:

- ☐ 1 cup frozen bananas, sliced
- ☐ 3 pitted Medjool dates
- ☐ 1 tablespoon dark chocolate
- ☐ ½ pitted medium avocado
- ☐ 5 mint leaves
- ☐ 1 tablespoon organic dark chocolate chips
- ☐ 1 cup coconut or almond milk, plain

Directions:

-Take all of the ingredients and throw them into a blender at high speed

-Blend this until it's all smoothed

-Serve it immediately

Nutritional info:

Calories: 303
Sodium: 86 mg
Carbs: 57g
Fat: 9g
Fiber: 8g
Protein: 3g

Strawberry Pineapple Smoothie

This is another refreshing and wonderful taste, and it's a great one if you love strawberries!

Ingredients:

- ☐ 2 cups pineapple chunks
- ☐ ½ cup Greek yogurt
- ☐ 1 ½ cups unsweetened almond milk
- ☐ 2 cups frozen strawberries

Directions:

-Take all of the ingredients and throw them in a blender

-Blend this on a high speed until smooth, adding milk as needed

-Serve with extra chunks of pineapple near the bottom

Nutritional information:

Calories: 165
Carbs: 30g
Fat: 2g
Protein: 8g
Fiber: 5g

Banana Matcha Smoothie

Matcha is great! And combined with bananas it makes a killer combination everyone will enjoy

Ingredients:

- ☐ 1 cup frozen bananas, sliced
- ☐ 1 cup packed spinach
- ☐ 1 teaspoon vanilla extract
- ☐ 1 teaspoon matcha powder
- ☐ 2 tablespoons flax seed
- ☐ 1 cup unsweetened almond milk

Directions:

-Take all of the ingredients and throw them into a blender until smoothed

Nutritional info:

Calories: 203
Fat: 5g

Carbs: 39g
Fiber: 6g
Protein: 4g

Plant Paradox Green Smoothie

This is one with a lot of green in it, and has a lot of great nutritional additives to this. In fact, it has way more veggies, and is a powerful green smoothie

Ingredients:

- ☐ 6 cups of chopped lettuce, romaine
- ☐ 1 avocado, ripe
- ☐ 1 small bunch of mint leaves and stems
- ☐ 3 cups baby spinach leaves
- ☐ 1 piece of raw ginger
- ☐ 3 tablespoons coconut butter
- ☐ 1 juiced lemon
- ☐ 3 cups of cold water

Directions:

-Chop, wash and measure the ingredients

-From here fill up the lettuce, then add in the other ingredients

-Add the water to the top, then blend it till it's high and smooth

-Taste, adding more water for thickness

-Serve! You'll get 3 servings out of this, so a lot to go around

Nutritional information:

Calories: 142
Fat: 4g
Protein: 5g
Fiber: 10g
Carbs: 22g

Purple Smoothie

This is another great smoothie option, especially if you're looking for dairy-free or vegan options

Ingredients:

- ☐   1 cup coconut or unsweetened almond milk
- ☐   ¼ cup coconut yogurt, left unsweetened
- ☐   ¼ cup purple sweet potato
- ☐   1 handful of baby spinach
- ☐   1 cup berries, frozen
- ☐   2 drops of liquid stevia

Directions:

-Put it all in a blender and mix it together, then serve

Nutritional information:

Calories: 115
Fat: 2g
Protein: 2g
Carbs: 12g
Sodium: 80mg

Strawberry Banana Smoothie

This is another great one if you're looking to make bagged lectins-free smoothies for those on-the-go moments.

Ingredients:

- ☐   2 cups frozen bananas
- ☐   4 cups frozen spinach
- ☐   2 cups strawberries
- ☐   4 teaspoons chia seeds

Directions:

-First you want to lay out the bananas, strawberries, and any other fruit you use on parchment paper, putting it in the fridge for 2 hours or until frozen

-Take freezer bags and then add a cup of the fruit, then the spinach, then the chia seeds

-Get the air out of the bags. When it's time to blend, put the contents into the blender

-Add about ½ a cup of milk and some protein powder

-Blend everything on high for a minute

Nutritional information:

Calories: 196
Fat: 4g
Carbs 23g
Fiber: 6g
Protein: 16g

10 Lunch Lectins-Free Smoothie Recipes

And now for lunch. This is another fun time to have all of the great smoothies that you can get. Since it's all lectins-free, they are simple, yet effective to have no matter what time of day you're taking your lunch.

Triple Berry Smoothie

Who doesn't love berries? Well now you can bring them on the go and during lunch with this amazing green smoothie

Ingredients:

- ☐ 1 ½ cups frozen berry mix
- ☐ ½ tablespoon chia seeds
- ☐ 2 cups unsweetened almond milk
- ☐ 1 medium banana, frozen
- ☐ ¼ cup vanilla powder that has protein

Directions:

-Take all of the ingredients, leaving half a cup of milk to the side and blend it

-Add more milk till it's smooth

Nutritional info:

Calories: 197
Fat: 3g
Fiber: 8g
Protein: 12g

Pumpkin Berry Smoothie

The refreshing taste of pumpkin can be indulged in with this fun smoothie! Here is a great lectins-free pumpkin smoothie

Ingredients:

- ☐ 2 tablespoons organic pumpkin puree
- ☐ 1 cup frozen blueberries
- ☐ ½ tablespoon flaxseed meal
- ☐ 1 cup unsweetened almond milk
- ☐ 1 tablespoon nut butter
- ☐ ½ a frozen banana
- ☐ ½ teaspoon pumpkin pie spice

Directions:

-Put all of the ingredients in a blender and blend till smoothed out

-Scrape and add more almond milk, blending till smooth

Nutritional info:

Calories: 288
Fat: 12g
Fiber: 9g
Protein: 7g
Carbs: 35g

Chocolate protein Shake

This is a filling, whole shake that's perfect for when you need something that has a lot of power, and perfect for those on-the-go meals

Ingredients:

- ☐ 1 cup frozen blueberries
- ☐ ¼ cup protein powder of choice, but chocolate flavored
- ☐ ¼ cup nonfat Greek yogurt
- ☐ ½ teaspoon ground flaxseed
- ☐ 1 medium banana, frozen
- ☐ 1 tablespoon organic cocoa powder
- ☐ 2 tablespoons nut butter
- ☐ 1 cup unsweetened almond milk

Directions:

-Put in blender and blend on high

-Scrape the sides after a minute, then blend till smooth

-Serve right then!

Nutritional info:

Calories: 280
Fat: 10g
Carbs: 36g
Fiber: 6g
Protein: 17g

Blueberry Banana Smoothie

A simple fruity smoothie, it's good for when you need something quick and on the go. Also good with a protein powder addition!

Ingredients:

- [ ] 1 cup frozen blueberries
- [ ] 1 tablespoon flax meal
- [ ] 1 teaspoon vanilla
- [ ] 1 cup frozen bananas, sliced
- [ ] 1 cup almond milk, unsweetened

Directions:

-Take all of the ingredients and then blend it till smooth

Nutritional info:

Calories: 147
Sodium: 92 mg
Fat: 3g
Carbs: 29g
Fiber: 5
Protein: 3g

Dark Chocolate date Smoothie

Another amazing protein smoothie. This one has 10 grams of protein and 9 grams of fiber, which is a great way to keep you full throughout the rest of the day, and energy to keep you going!

Ingredients:

- [ ] 2 medium bananas
- [ ] 1 cup deboned and chopped kale
- [ ] 3 pitted dates

- ☐ ½ teaspoon vanilla extract
- ☐ 3 tablespoons cocoa powder
- ☐ 1 cup nut milk

Directions:

-Take all of the ingredients and blend it till smoothed out

-If you like a thicker smoothie, you can always put more nut milk in

Nutritional info:

Calories: 312
Sodium: 213 mg
Fat: 6g
Carbs: 65g
Fiber: 9g
Protein: 10g

Strawberry Chia Seed Smoothie

A simple smoothie, but this one contains both strawberries which are great, some filling Greek yogurt, and some chia seeds.

Ingredients:

- ☐ 1 cup frozen strawberries
- ☐ ½ cup plain Greek yogurt
- ☐ ½ cup vanilla extract
- ☐ 1 medium banana
- ☐ 1 cup unsweetened almond milk
- ☐ 1 tablespoon of chia seeds

Directions:

-Take all of the ingredients and blend it till smoothed out

-Let the chia seeds expand before you drink it

Nutritional info:

Calories: 159
Sodium: 102 mg
Fat: 3g
Carbs: 24g
Fiber: 5g
Protein: 9g

Apple Pie Smoothie

This can be done either as a smoothie itself, or as a smoothie bowl. It is sweet, and really good

Ingredients:

- ☐ 1 frozen banana, kept small
- ☐ ½ cup organic apples
- ☐ 1 teaspoon cinnamon
- ☐ ½ cup unsweetened almond milk
- ☐ ½ cup nonfat vanilla Greek yogurt
- ☐ ¼ cup rolled oats
- ☐ 1 teaspoon vanilla extract
- ☐ A handful of leafy greens of choice

Directions:

-Take the apples ae chop them up to smaller pieces

-Put all of the ingredients together into a blender, and then blend it all until smooth

-If you decide to make it a smoothie bowl, you can add fixings, or even just top the
smoothie with little fixings of choice

-You can take out the Greek yogurt and add almond milk too

Nutritional info:

Calories: 328
Carbs: 52
Fiber: 9g
Protein: 17g
Fat: 3g

Kale Smoothie

Leafy greens are a staple of the lectins-free diet, but for some, it gets a bit tiresome after a while. Well, here's an amazing smoothie made with kale to really stimulate your taste buds

Ingredients:

- ☐ 2 cups bananas, frozen
- ☐ 1 tablespoon flax meal
- ☐ ½ teaspoon fresh grated ginger
- ☐ 2 cups packed chopped kale

☐ 2 pitted medjool dates
☐ 1 cup of oranges, juiced

Directions:

-Take all of the ingredients and throw it into a blender

-Blend it on high until smoothed

-Serve with toppings if you desire

Nutritional info:

Calories: 226
Fat: 2g
Carbs: 50g
Fiber: 6g
Protein: 5g

Apple Smoothie

Apples are a great ingredient added to many smoothies. Here is a fun, simple apple smoothie that's great for you.

Ingredients:

☐ 1 cup unsweetened nut milk of choice
☐ 1 cup apples, sliced
☐ 1 teaspoon cinnamon
☐ 1 teaspoon nutmeg
☐ A handful of kale
☐ Protein powder of choice

Directions:

-Take all of the ingredients and then blend this until smoothed

Nutrition facts:

Calories: 220
Fat: 4g
Protein: 16
Carbs: 30g
Sodium: 100mg

Milky Mango Smoothie

This does have a natural nut milk in it, and it all comes together to give you a wonderful smoothie that's made with a lot of love, and a lot of natural ingredients. Perfect for those looking for a supplemental, amazing smoothie that they can rely on.

Ingredients:

- ☐ 1 tablespoon of turmeric, which has amazing health benefits
- ☐ 1 cup Greek yogurt or nut milk
- ☐ 1 cup frozen mango
- ☐ 1 frozen banana, sliced, or 1 cup of sliced cauliflower
- ☐ Splash of water to help really smooth it out

Directions:

-Take all of the ingredients and blend it

-Add more nut milk if you've got some and want to make it thicker

Nutritional info:

Calories: 270
Fat: 1g
Sodium: 75 mg
Carbs: 60g
Protein: 18g

10 Dinner Lectins-Free Smoothie Recipes

And now there's dinner. There's a lot to prepare for dinner, and a lot that you can do to really make your smoothies for dinner better than ever!

Lectin-Free Green Smoothie

This is a simple green smoothie that comes with a lot of great items. It's pretty simple, and sweet, and it can help with a low-calorie option for those looking for an additive for dinner. It also is good if you want to safely reduce your calorie intake, and can help to suppress your appetite too.

Ingredients:

- ☐ 2 cups unsweetened almond milk

☐   ½ of a small avocado
☐   1 tablespoon ground flaxseeds
☐   1 cup of ice cubes
☐   2 cups fresh spinach
☐   4 mint leaves, fresh
☐   6 drops of stevia

Directions:

-Add all of the ingredients and blend it together

-If you want to have a bit more sweetness, you can put ½ a green apple in there

Nutritional info:

Calories: 140
Fat: 4g
Carbs: 22g
Protein: 7g
Sodium: 82 mg

Lectin-Free Chocolate Smoothie

For those of us who have a sweet tooth for chocolate, this is another fun chocolate smoothie. It is lectins-free and has a few ingredients. This also can help with your heart health and weight loss, and with the addition of stevia, it's a fun smoothie and doesn't have a huge aftertaste either. You can add monk fruit too for more anti-inflammatory benefits

Ingredients:

☐   2 cups unsweetened nut milk
☐   6 drops of stevia, vanilla
☐   ½ an avocado
☐   1 tablespoon hemp seeds
☐   2 tablespoons organic raw cocoa powder
☐   ½ of a monk fruit (optional)

Directions:

-Take all of the ingredients and blend them all together until properly smooth

-For a more refreshing taste, you can add some ice to this to really make the smoothie strong

Nutritional info:

Calories: 220
Fat: 3g
Protein: 7g
Carbs: 23g

Banana Mango Smoothie

This is another sweet and refreshing smoothie. It is best topped with hemp seeds too if that's something that you enjoy.

Ingredients:

- ☐ 1 banana, sliced
- ☐ 3 handfuls of spinach or baby kale
- ☐ ½ a cup of unsweetened almond milk
- ☐ A handful of ice
- ☐ ½ a diced mango
- ☐ 2 tablespoons of hemp seeds
- ☐ 1/8 of a teaspoon of pink salt

Directions:

-Take all of the ingredients, throw them into a blender

-Process this until it's totally smooth

-Put the smoothie into the bowl and add toppings of choice such as hemp seeds, raw honey or kale sprouts

Nutritional info:

Calories: 215
Carbs: 25g
Fat: 4g
Protein: 6g

Strawberry Pomegranate Green Smoothie

This is a cool smoothie because not only does it have a lot of amazing antioxidant-fruits, but also it has two fun layers, which offer a lot of health benefits. This is just a fun smoothie, and really good as well if you like the refreshing taste of coconut

Ingredients:

- ☐ 1 frozen banana of choice
- ☐ ½ a cup of coconut water
- ☐ 1 cup frozen strawberries

- ☐ A sprig of mint
- ☐ (for the green layer)
- ☐ 1 cup of fresh spinach
- ☐ ¼ cup pomegranates
- ☐ ½ a frozen banana
- ☐ ¼ cup coconut water

Directions:

-Begin with the top ingredients first, putting them into a blender and blend it until smoothed

-Pour it in a mason jar, then clean your blender, adding the green layer ingredients to this. Blend it till properly mixed

-You can add a scoop of protein powder as well if you'd like to include a protein additive to this

Nutritional info:

Calories: 158
Carbs: 32g
Fat: 4g
Fiber: 10g
Protein: 6g

Carrot Cake Smoothie

Carrot cake is an indulging dessert, and lots of people do enjoy it. Well now you can have it at the convenience of a fun, refreshing smoothie. Not only that, but it has also far fewer calories compared to this too!

Ingredients:

- ☐ 8 walnuts
- ☐ Grated carrot to mix in
- ☐ Sprinkle of nutmeg
- ☐ 1 cup of nut milk
- ☐ ½ a frozen banana
- ☐ 1 teaspoon of cinnamon
- ☐ 2 dates, pitted
- ☐ 1 teaspoon vanilla

Directions:

-Take all of the ingredients and then blend this together minus the carrot until it's smooth and creamy

-Mix in the carrot with the rest of it

-Add a couple of walnuts to the top if that's what you like, and then you can enjoy it!

-If you're looking for a better alternative to walnuts, use almonds

Nutritional info:

Calories: 260
Fat: 8g
Protein: 10g
Fiber: 14g
Carbs: 42g

Snickerdoodle Green Smoothie

This is a sweet, fun smoothie that's great if you want a sweet little dessert smoothie, but also lectins-free. It also works well with vanilla protein powder, so if you want to throw a scoop or two into there, then go for it.

Ingredients:

- ☐ A handful of spinach
- ☐ ½ a small avocado
- ☐ ½ a teaspoon of vanilla
- ☐ 1 frozen banana
- ☐ ¼ cup of unsweetened almond milk
- ☐ ¼ teaspoon cinnamon
- ☐ Protein powder (optional)

Directions:

-Take all of the ingredients and blend them together

-Serve!

Nutritional info:

Calories: 152
Protein: 10g
Fat: 5g
Carbs: 20g

Green Warrior Smoothie

Talk about a protein meal in a glass. This is great if you want high-protein sources but also a ton of fiber and fatty acids too. This is great for cravings as well.

Ingredients:

- ☐ ½ a cup of red grapefruit, juiced
- ☐ 1 large cored and chopped apple
- ☐ 1 large celery stalk, chopped
- ☐ 1 cup of baby spinach
- ☐ 1 cup of chopped cucumber
- ☐ 3 tablespoons of hemp hearts
- ☐ 2 tablespoons packed mint leaves
- ☐ Ice cubes as needed
- ☐ ½ cup of frozen mango
- ☐ 2 tablespoons virgin coconut oil

Directions:

-Juice your grapefruit and put it in the blender

-Add in all of the other ingredients, adding more ice as needed

-Blend it all together, adding more water as needed, and then serve it immediately!

-You can add the leftovers to the fridge if you want to have it left over

Nutritional info:

Calories: 220
Fat: 10g
Carbs: 30g
Protein: 14g
Fiber: 10g

Leprechaun Smoothie

This is a higher-calorie smoothie, but it has a lot of great options added to it, that's perfect for those nights when you just want to have something that'll keep you full for the duration of the evening. It is similar to a shamrock shake, but it doesn't include a bunch of sugar, and has many more healthy additions, and is really good if you want something that's low in carbs, while also really packed with other amazing nutrients.

Ingredients:

- ☐ ½ an avocado

- ☐ ¼ cup fresh spinach
- ☐ ¼ cup vanilla or plain whey protein, or egg protein
- ☐ ¼ cup coconut milk or heavy whipping cream
- ☐ Mint extract or a mint sprig
- ☐ 2 tablespoons almonds or pistachio nuts
- ☐ Seeds from a vanilla bean or a teaspoon of vanilla extract
- ☐ 5 drops liquid stevia
- ☐ ½ a cup of water or some ice cubes

Directions:

-Take the mint and spinach and wash them, then peel the avocado.

-Blend all of these together till smooth, then add in the other ingredients

-Serve it immediately!

Nutritional info:

Calories: 493
Carbs: 9g
Protein: 27g
Fat: 37g
Fiber: 14g

Purple Power Smoothie

Purple smoothies are really good since they contain lectins-free starches that are healthy for you. This contains a lot of superfoods within it, and it's all neatly packed together to create the best smoothie that you can have, and one that's worth indulging in, no matter what.

This also contains an array of different antioxidants, which are wonderful for your health as well.

Ingredients:

- ☐ ½ cup of coconut water nut milk, or regular water
- ☐ ½ cup of frozen strawberries
- ☐ 1 teaspoon acai powder
- ☐ ½ cup frozen cherries
- ☐ ¼ cup frozen blueberries
- ☐ Protein powder to add in
- ☐ Nut butter to add in
- ☐ Milled flaxseed to add in
- ☐ Handful of spinach
- ☐ Maca powder as an add-in

Directions:

-Take all of the ingredients and put this into a blender

-For smaller blenders, you want to put the last five ingredients in there at the end

-Blend this till smoothed, then add the ingredients, and then blend it together to create the perfect consistency for this

Nutritional info:

Calories: 230
Fat: 5g
Sodium: 15mg
Carbs: 25g
Fiber: 8g
Protein: 15g

Oatmeal Smoothie

Finally, we have this refreshing oatmeal smoothie. Oats are really good for feeling full, and good for an array of different health benefits. In this, we'll go over some of the amazing ingredients within this simple smoothie, and how an oatmeal smoothie is perfect for every time of the day

Ingredients:

- ¼ cup old-fashioned oats or quick oats
- ½ cup unsweetened almond milk
- 1.2 tablespoon pure maple syrup
- ½ teaspoon ground cinnamon
- 1 chopped banana
- 1 tablespoon nut butter
- ½ teaspoon vanilla extract
- 1/8 teaspoon kosher salt
- Optional ice

Directions:

-Take the oats and put them at the bottom of your blender, blending until grounded

-Put the rest of the ingredients into there and blend it until it's smoothed out

-Add more stevia if you're looking for a smoothie which is sweeter

-Serve this immediately!

Don't be Afraid to Mix-In Additives

One big thing people need to remember with these smoothies is they're a good way to start. In fact, this should be the springboard that they go off of. With that being said, if you want to add more protein and such to the mix, don't be afraid to do so.

Mix-ins are great because they offer additives in terms of nutrition. Most of these are low-calorie, so if you start to notice that you're feeling like you need something more added to that, then you should definitely consider adding a protein supplement to this.

You can also add other additives too. Matcha powder for example has a ton of antioxidants to this. Agave syrup is another popular additive to add as well.

Another very popular one too is raw honey. Raw honey has amazing benefits, and it can be used to naturally sweeten any smoothie, so if you notice that you require a better smoothie and a sweeter taste, then definitely consider adding this.

As for how to do this smoothie diet, consider making smoothies, use them, and see how you feel. For some people, moving towards the smoothie diet is easy, especially if you didn't have a super active lifestyle before all of this.

If you notice you're getting very hungry though, don't be afraid to incorporate more calories to your foods. That way you can stay fuller for longer. You should make sure to do what works for you in terms of these smoothies.

Remember you can always substitute out these fruits too. If you're not a fan of bananas for example, substituting them with another superfruit may be another great thing for you to do. Also, incorporating more dark, leafy greens is another great option especially if you want something that's filling, and something that contains a variety of different antioxidants.

You can also make these smoothies and grab and go. We discussed the bag smoothies as well, so if that's what you're looking to incorporate, consider doing that.

Finally, we did mention the smoothie bowls. This is essentially a smoothie itself, but put in a bowl form. While this isn't for everyone, this is definitely something to consider if you're bored with the current smoothies that you have, and you want something a little bit different for your palate as well.

And there you have it, some lectins-free smoothies to try out and choose from. If you've ever been curious about lectins-free smoothies, then this is one of the best places to start. They are good, wholesome, and filling, which is perfect for anyone looking to really get the most out of their smoothie experience, no matter what it may be.

Conclusion

There you have it.

Everything you need to know about the lectins-free diet, and some amazing smoothies that can help you achieve the lectins-free lifestyle.

While this is a bit of a different diet than what most of us are used to, it's a good idea to get into eating better, and reducing the inflammation in the body.

While it may be hard to really keep up with it for the duration, it does propose a healthier lifestyle, and if you know that your body is reactive towards lectins, then you should make sure that you do something about it, since it can affect you in a negative manner.

With that being said, try these smoothies today, see the difference it makes, and don't be afraid to experiment with all of this, since there are plenty of options for you to choose from!

Thank You

Thank you for buying my book and I hope you enjoyed it. If you found any value in this book I would really appreciate it if you'd take a minute to post a review about this book. I check all my reviews and love to get feedback.

This is the real reward for me knowing that I'm helping others. If you know anyone who may enjoy this book, please share the message and gift it to them.

About Author

Nicole Gibbs holds a science degree in nutrition and is clinically trained in all areas of nutrition. In addition to her twenty year's experience in the field of nutrition, she also has a culinary background as well as a passion and desire for making a difference in other people's lives through her work.

Nicole Gibbs has written any books deepening and expanding what is already a wealth of knowledge. She is passionate and truly loves what she does and is driven by the success she has helped others achieve.